MW00781074

MEDITERRANEAN DIET SIDE DISHES

LEARN HOW TO COOK MEDITERRANEAN THROUGH THIS DETAILED COOKBOOK,
COMPLETE OF SEVERAL TASTY IDEAS FOR GOOD AND HEALTY SIDE DISHES.
SUITABLE FOT BOYTH ADULTS AND KIDS, IT WILL HELP YOU LOSE WEIGHT AND
FEEL BETTER, WITHOUT GIVING UP YOUR FAVOURITE FOOD

Table of Contents

Balsamic Baby Carrots

Prep time: 10 minutes I **Cooking time:** 40 minutes I **Servings:** 4

Ingredients:
- 1 pound baby carrots, peeled
- 1 tablespoon olive oil
- 2 spring onions, chopped
- 2 tablespoons balsamic vinegar
- 2 garlic cloves, minced
- 1 teaspoon turmeric powder
- 1 tablespoon chives, chopped
- ¼ teaspoon cayenne pepper
- A pinch of salt and black pepper

Directions:
1. Spread the carrots on a baking sheet lined with parchment paper, add the oil, the spring onions and the other ingredients, toss and bake at 380 degrees F for 40 minutes.
2. Divide the carrots between plates and serve.

Nutrition facts per serving: calories 79, fat 3.8, fiber 3.7, carbs 10.9, protein 1

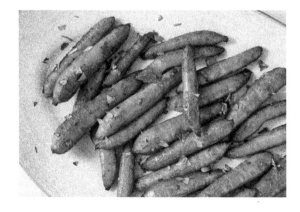

Paprika Spinach

Prep time: 10 minutes I **Cooking time:** 12 minutes I **Servings:** 4

Ingredients:
- 1 pound baby spinach
- 1 yellow onion, chopped
- 1 tablespoon olive oil
- 1 tablespoon lemon juice
- 2 garlic cloves, minced
- A pinch of cayenne pepper
- ¼ teaspoon smoked paprika
- A pinch of salt and black pepper

Directions:
1. Heat up a pan with the oil over medium-high heat, add the onion and the garlic and sauté for 2 minutes.
2. Add the spinach and the other ingredients, toss, cook over medium heat for 10 minutes, divide between plates and serve as a side dish.

Nutrition facts per serving: calories 71, fat 4, fiber 3.2, carbs 7.4, protein 3.7

Rosemary Carrots and Onion Mix

Prep time: 5 minutes I **Cooking time:** 25 minutes I **Servings:** 4

Ingredients:
- 1 pound carrots, peeled and roughly sliced
- 1 yellow onion, chopped
- 1 tablespoon olive oil
- Zest of 1 orange, grated
- Juice of 1 orange
- 1 orange, peeled and cut into segments
- 1 tablespoon rosemary, chopped
- A pinch of salt and black pepper

Directions:
1. Heat up a pan with the oil over medium-high heat, add the onion and sauté for 5 minutes.
2. Add the carrots, the orange zest and the other ingredients, toss, cook over medium heat for 20 minutes more, divide between plates and serve.

Nutrition facts per serving: calories 140, fat 3.9, fiber 5, carbs 26.1, protein 2.1

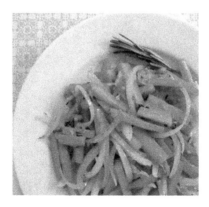

Endives and Scallions Sauté

Prep time: 5 minutes I **Cooking time:** 15 minutes I **Servings:** 4

Ingredients:
- 3 endives, shredded
- 1 tablespoon olive oil
- 4 scallions, chopped
- ½ cup tomato sauce
- 2 garlic cloves, minced
- A pinch of sea salt and black pepper
- 1/8 teaspoon turmeric powder
- 1 tablespoon chives, chopped

Directions:
1. Heat up a pan with the oil over medium heat, add the scallions and the garlic and sauté for 5 minutes.
2. Add the endives and the other ingredients, toss, cook everything for 10 minutes more, divide between plates and serve as a side dish.

Nutrition facts per serving: calories 110, fat 4.4, fiber 12.8, carbs 16.2, protein 5.6

Zucchini and Apples Mix

Prep time: 5 minutes I **Cooking time:** 20 minutes I **Servings:** 4

Ingredients:
- 1 pound zucchinis, sliced
- 1 yellow onion, chopped
- 2 tablespoons olive oil
- 2 apples, peeled, cored and cubed
- 1 tomato, cubed
- 1 tablespoon rosemary, chopped
- 1 tablespoon chives, chopped

Directions:
1. Heat up a pan with the oil over medium heat, add the onion and sauté for 5 minutes.
2. Add the zucchinis and the other ingredients, toss, cook over medium heat for 15 minutes more, divide between plates and serve as a side dish.

Nutrition facts per serving: calories 170, fat 5, fiber 2, carbs 11, protein 7

Balsamic Lime Mushrooms

Prep time: 10 minutes I **Cooking time:** 20 minutes I **Servings:** 4

Ingredients:
- 1 pound mushrooms, sliced
- 1 yellow onion, chopped
- 1 tablespoon ginger, grated
- 1 tablespoon olive oil
- 2 tablespoons balsamic vinegar
- 2 garlic cloves, minced
- A pinch of salt and black pepper
- ¼ cup lime juice
- 2 tablespoons walnuts, chopped

Directions:
1. Heat up a pan with the oil over medium-high heat, add the onion and the ginger and sauté for 5 minutes.
2. Add the mushrooms and the other ingredients, toss, cook over medium heat for 15 minutes more, divide between plates and serve.

Nutrition facts per serving: calories 120, fat 2, fiber 2, carbs 4, protein 5

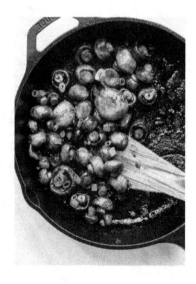

Bell Peppers and Scallions Mix

Prep time: 5 minutes I **Cooking time:** 20 minutes I **Servings:** 4

Ingredients:
- 1 red bell pepper, cut into strips
- 1 yellow bell pepper, cut into strips
- 1 green bell pepper, cut into strips
- 1 orange bell pepper, cut into strips
- 3 scallions, chopped
- 1 tablespoon olive oil
- 1 tablespoon coconut aminos
- A pinch of salt and black pepper
- 1 tablespoon parsley, chopped
- 1 tablespoon rosemary, chopped

Directions:
1. Heat up a pan with the oil over medium-high heat, add the scallions and sauté for 5 minutes.
2. Add the bell peppers and the other ingredients, toss, cook over medium heat for 15 minutes more, divide between plates and serve.

Nutrition facts per serving: calories 120, fat 1, fiber 2, carbs 7, protein 6

Balsamic Kale

Prep time: 5 minutes I **Cooking time:** 20 minutes I **Servings:** 4

Ingredients:
- 1 cup cherry tomatoes, halved
- 1 pound baby kale
- 1 yellow onion, chopped
- 2 tablespoons olive oil
- 1 tablespoon balsamic vinegar
- 1 tablespoon cilantro, chopped
- 2 tablespoons vegetable stock
- A pinch of salt and black pepper

Directions:
1. Heat up a pan with the oil over medium heat, add the onion and sauté for 5 minutes.
2. Add the kale, tomatoes and the other ingredients, toss, cook over medium heat for 15 minutes more, divide between plates and serve as a side dish.

Nutrition facts per serving: calories 170, fat 6, fiber 6, carbs 9, protein 4

Paprika Artichokes

Prep time: 10 minutes I **Cooking time:** 25 minutes I **Servings:** 4

Ingredients:
- 2 artichokes, trimmed and halved
- 1 teaspoon chili powder
- 2 green chilies, mined
- 2 tablespoons olive oil
- 1 teaspoon garlic powder
- 1 teaspoon sweet paprika
- A pinch of salt and black pepper
- Juice of 1 lime

Directions:
1. In a roasting pan, combine the artichokes with the chili powder, the chilies and the other ingredients, toss and bake at 380 degrees F for 25 minutes.
2. Divide the artichokes between plates and serve.

Nutrition facts per serving: calories 132, fat 2, fiber 2, carbs 4, protein 6

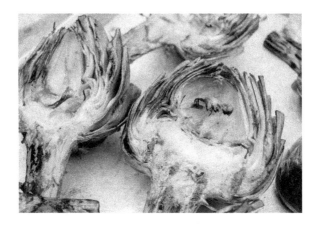

Ginger Sprouts

Prep time: 10 minutes I **Cooking time:** 20 minutes I **Servings:** 4

Ingredients:
- 2 tablespoons olive oil
- 1 pound Brussels sprouts, trimmed and halved
- 1 tablespoon ginger, grated
- 2 garlic cloves, minced
- 1 tablespoon pine nuts
- 1 tablespoon olive oil

Directions:
1. Heat up a pan with the oil over medium heat, add the garlic and the ginger and sauté for 2 minutes.
2. Add the Brussels sprouts and the other ingredients, toss, cook for 18 minutes more, divide between plates and serve.

Nutrition facts per serving: calories 160, fat 2, fiber 2, carbs 4, protein 5

Paprika Cauliflower

Prep time: 10 minutes I **Cooking time:** 25 minutes I **Servings:** 4

Ingredients:
- 1 pound cauliflower florets
- 2 tablespoons avocado oil
- 1 teaspoon nutmeg, ground
- 1 teaspoon hot paprika
- 1 tablespoon pumpkin seeds
- 1 tablespoon chives, chopped
- A pinch of sea salt and black pepper

Directions:
1. Spread the cauliflower florets on a baking sheet lined with parchment paper, add the oil, the nutmeg and the other ingredients, toss and bake at 380 degrees F for 25 minutes.
2. Divide the cauliflower mix between plates and serve as a side dish.

Nutrition facts per serving: calories 160, fat 3, fiber 2, carbs 9, protein 4

Garlic Broccoli

Prep time: 10 minutes I **Cooking time:** 30 minutes I **Servings:** 4

Ingredients:
- 2 tablespoons olive oil
- 1 pound broccoli florets
- 1 tablespoon garlic, minced
- 1 tablespoon pine nuts, toasted
- 1 tablespoon lemon juice
- 2 teaspoons mustard
- A pinch of salt and black pepper

Directions:
1. In a roasting pan, combine the broccoli with the oil, the garlic and the other ingredients, toss and bake at 380 degrees F for 30 minutes.
2. Divide everything between plates and serve as a side dish.

Nutrition facts per serving: calories 220, fat 6, fiber 2, carbs 7, protein 6

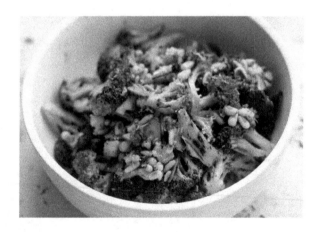

Cilantro Quinoa

Prep time: 10 minutes I **Cooking time:** 30 minutes I **Servings:** 4

Ingredients:
- 1 yellow onion, chopped
- 1 tomato, cubed
- 1 cup quinoa
- 3 cups vegetable stock
- 1 tablespoon olive oil
- 1 cup peas
- 1 tablespoon cilantro, chopped
- A pinch of salt and black pepper

Directions:
1. Heat up a pot with the oil over medium heat, add the onion, stir and sauté for 5 minutes.
2. Add the quinoa, the stock and the other ingredients, toss, bring to a simmer and cook over medium heat for 25 minutes.
3. Divide everything between plates and serve as a side dish.

Nutrition facts per serving: calories 202, fat 3, fiber 3, carbs 11, protein 6

Green Beans and Sauce

Prep time: 10 minutes I **Cooking time:** 20 minutes I **Servings:** 4

Ingredients:
- 1 yellow onion, chopped
- 1 pound green beans, trimmed and halved
- 1 tablespoon avocado oil
- 2 teaspoons basil, dried
- A pinch of salt and black pepper
- 1 tablespoon tomato sauce

Directions:
1. Heat up a pan with the oil over medium-high heat, add the onion and sauté for 5 minutes.
2. Add the green beans and the other ingredients, toss, cook for 15 minutes more.
3. Divide everything between plates and serve as a side dish.

Nutrition facts per serving: calories 221, fat 5, fiber 8, carbs 10, protein 8

Garlic Brussels Sprouts

Prep time: 10 minutes I **Cooking time:** 20 minutes I **Servings:** 4

Ingredients:
- 2 pounds Brussels sprouts, trimmed and halved
- 1 tablespoon avocado oil
- 2 tablespoons balsamic vinegar
- 3 garlic cloves, minced
- 1 tablespoon cilantro, chopped
- A pinch of salt and black pepper

Directions:
1. Heat up a pan with the oil over medium-high heat, add the garlic and sauté for 2 minutes.
2. Add the sprouts and the other ingredients, toss, cook over medium heat for 18 minutes more, divide between plates and serve.

Nutrition facts per serving: calories 108, fat 1.2, fiber 8.7, carbs 21.7, protein 7.9

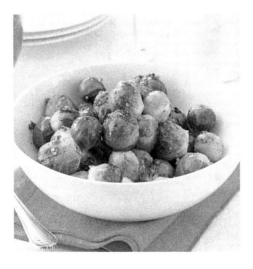

Chives Cabbage

Prep time: 10 minutes I **Cooking time:** 20 minutes I **Servings:** 4

Ingredients:
- 1 green cabbage head, shredded
- 1 yellow onion, chopped
- 1 beet, peeled and cubed
- ½ cup chicken stock
- 2 tablespoons olive oil
- A pinch of salt and black pepper
- 2 tablespoons chives, chopped

Directions:
1. Heat up a pan with the oil over medium heat, add the onion and sauté for 5 minutes.
2. Add the cabbage and the other ingredients, toss, cook over medium heat for 15 minutes more, divide between plates and serve.

Nutrition facts per serving: calories 128, fat 7.3, fiber 5.6, carbs 15.6, protein 3.1

Garlic Asparagus Saute

Prep time: 10 minutes I **Cooking time:** 15 minutes I **Servings:** 4

Ingredients:
- 1 yellow onion, chopped
- 2 tablespoons olive oil
- 1 bunch asparagus, trimmed and halved
- 2 garlic cloves, minced
- 1 teaspoon chili powder
- ¼ cup cilantro, chopped

Directions:
1. Heat up a pan with the oil over medium-high heat, add the onion and the garlic and sauté for 5 minutes.
2. Add the asparagus and the other ingredients, toss, cook for 10 minutes, divide between plates and serve.

Nutrition facts per serving: calories 80, fat 7.2, fiber 1.4, carbs 4.4, protein 1

Turmeric Quinoa

Prep time: 10 minutes I **Cooking time:** 25 minutes I **Servings:** 4

Ingredients:
- 1 cup quinoa
- 3 cups chicken stock
- 1 cup tomatoes, cubed
- 1 tablespoon parsley, chopped
- 1 tablespoon basil, chopped
- 1 teaspoon turmeric powder
- A pinch of salt and black pepper

Directions:
1. In a pot, mix the quinoa with the stock, the tomatoes and the other ingredients, toss, bring to a simmer and cook over medium heat for 25 minutes.
2. Divide everything between plates and serve.

Nutrition facts per serving: calories 202, fat 4, fiber 2, carbs 12, protein 10

Black Beans and Peppers Mix

Prep time: 10 minutes I **Cooking time:** 20 minutes I **Servings:** 4

Ingredients:
- 1 tablespoon olive oil
- 2 cups black beans, cooked and drained
- 1 green bell pepper, chopped
- 1 yellow onion, chopped
- 4 garlic cloves, minced
- 1 teaspoon cumin, ground
- ½ cup chicken stock
- 1 tablespoon coriander, chopped
- A pinch of salt and black pepper

Directions:
1. Heat up a pan with the oil over medium heat, add the onion and the garlic and sauté for 5 minutes.
2. Add the black beans and the other ingredients, toss, cook over medium heat for 15 minutes more, divide between plates and serve.

Nutrition facts per serving: calories 221, fat 5, fiber 4, carbs 9, protein 11

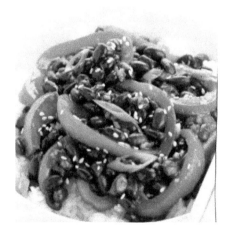

Oregano Green Beans

Prep time: 10 minutes I **Cooking time:** 20 minutes I **Servings:** 4

Ingredients:
- 1 pound green beans, trimmed and halved
- 3 scallions, chopped
- 1 mango, peeled and cubed
- 2 tablespoons olive oil
- ½ cup veggie stock
- 1 tablespoon oregano, chopped
- 1 teaspoon sweet paprika
- A pinch of salt and black pepper

Directions:
1. Heat up a pan with the oil over medium heat, add the scallions and sauté for 2 minutes.
2. Add the green beans and the other ingredients, toss, cook over medium heat for 18 minutes more, divide between plates and serve.

Nutrition facts per serving: calories 182, fat 4, fiber 5, carbs 6, protein 8

Quinoa with Green Onions

Prep time: 10 minutes I **Cooking time:** 30 minutes I **Servings:** 4

Ingredients:
- 1 yellow onion, chopped
- 1 tablespoon olive oil
- 1 cup quinoa
- 3 cups vegetable stock
- ½ cup black olives, pitted and halved
- 2 green onions, chopped
- 2 tablespoons coconut aminos
- 1 teaspoon rosemary, dried

Directions:
1. Heat up a pot with the oil over medium heat, add the yellow onion and sauté for 5 minutes.
2. Add the quinoa and the other ingredients except the green onions, stir, bring to a simmer and cook over medium heat for 25 minutes.
3. Divide the mix between plates, sprinkle the green onions on top and serve.

Nutrition facts per serving: calories 261, fat 6, fiber 8, carbs 10, protein 6

Coconut Potato Mash

Prep time: 10 minutes I **Cooking time:** 25 minutes I **Servings:** 4

Ingredients:
- 1 cup veggie stock
- 1 pound sweet potatoes, peeled and cubed
- 1 cup coconut cream
- 2 teaspoons olive oil
- A pinch of salt and black pepper
- ½ teaspoon turmeric powder
- 1 tablespoon chives, chopped

Directions:
1. In a pot, combine the stock with the sweet potatoes and the other ingredients except the cream, the oil and the chives, stir, bring to a simmer and cook over medium heat fro 25 minutes.
2. Add the rest of the ingredients, mash the mix well, stir it, divide between plates and serve.

Nutrition facts per serving: calories 200, fat 4, fiber 4, carbs 7, protein 10

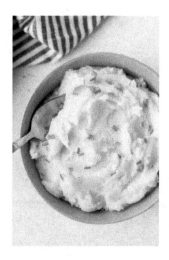

Coconut Peas

Prep time: 10 minutes I **Cooking time:** 20 minutes I **Servings:** 4

Ingredients:
- 1 cup coconut cream
- 1 yellow onion, chopped
- 1 tablespoon olive oil
- 2 cups green peas
- A pinch of salt and black pepper
- A pinch of salt and black pepper

Directions:
1. Heat up a pan with the oil over medium heat, add the onion and sauté for 5 minutes.
2. Add the peas and the other ingredients, toss, cook over medium heat for 15 minutes, divide between plates and serve.

Nutrition facts per serving: calories 191, fat 5, fiber 4, carbs 11, protein 9

Mushrooms Saute

Prep time: 10 minutes I **Cooking time:** 25 minutes I **Servings:** 4

Ingredients:
- 1 pound mushrooms, sliced
- 1 yellow onion, chopped
- 1 teaspoon cumin, ground
- 1 teaspoon sweet paprika
- 1 cup black beans, cooked
- 2 tablespoons olive oil
- ½ cup chicken stock
- A pinch of salt and black pepper
- 2 tablespoons cilantro, chopped

Directions:
1. Heat up a pan with the oil over medium heat, add the onion and sauté for 5 minutes.
2. Add the mushrooms and sauté for 5 minutes more.
3. Add the rest of the ingredients, toss, cook over medium heat for 15 minutes more.
4. Divide everything between plates and serve as a side dish.

Nutrition facts per serving: calories 189, fat 3, fiber 4, carbs 9, protein 8

Ginger Broccoli and Sprouts

Prep time: 10 minutes I **Cooking time:** 25 minutes I **Servings:** 4

Ingredients:
- 1 pound broccoli florets
- ½ pound Brussels sprouts, trimmed and halved
- 2 tablespoons olive oil
- 1 tablespoon ginger, grated
- 1 tablespoon balsamic vinegar
- A pinch of salt and black pepper

Directions:
1. In a roasting pan, combine the broccoli with the sprouts and the other ingredients, toss gently and bake at 380 degrees F for 25 minutes.
2. Divide the mix between plates and serve.

Nutrition facts per serving: calories 129, fat 7.6, fiber 5.3, carbs 13.7, protein 5.2

Maple Cauliflower

Prep time: 10 minutes I **Cooking time:** 25 minutes I **Servings:** 4

Ingredients:
- 1 tablespoon olive oil
- 1 pound cauliflower florets
- 1 tablespoon maple syrup
- 1 tablespoon rosemary, chopped
- A pinch of salt and black pepper
- 1 teaspoon chili powder

Directions:
1. Spread the cauliflower on a baking sheet lined with parchment paper, add the oil and the other ingredients, toss and cook in the oven at 375 degrees F for 25 minutes.
2. Divide the mix between plates and serve.

Nutrition facts per serving: calories 76, fat 3.9, fiber 3.4, carbs 10.3, protein 2.4

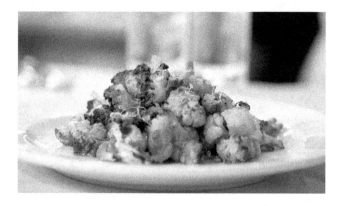

Turmeric Asparagus

Prep time: 10 minutes I **Cooking time:** 20 minutes I**Servings:** 4

Ingredients:
- 1 pound asparagus, trimmed and halved
- ½ pound cherry tomatoes, halved
- 2 tablespoons olive oil
- 1 teaspoon turmeric powder
- 2 tablespoons shallot, chopped
- A pinch of salt and black pepper
- 1 tablespoon chives, chopped

Directions:
1. Spread the asparagus on a baking sheet lined with parchment paper, add the tomatoes and the other ingredients, toss, cook in the oven at 375 degrees F for 20 minutes.
2. Divide everything between plates and serve as a side dish.

Nutrition facts per serving: calories 132, fat 1, fiber 2, carbs 4, protein 4

Chili and Dill Cucumber Mix

Prep time: 10 minutes I **Cooking time:** 0 minutes I **Servings:** 4

Ingredients:
- 1 pound cucumbers, sliced
- 1 tablespoon olive oil
- 1 teaspoon chili powder
- 1 green chili, chopped
- 1 garlic clove, minced
- 1 tablespoon dill, chopped
- 2 tablespoons lime juice
- 1 tablespoon balsamic vinegar

Directions:
1. In a bowl, combine the cucumbers with the garlic, the oil and the other ingredients, toss and serve as a side salad.

Nutrition facts per serving: calories 132, fat 3, fiber 1, carbs 7, protein 4

Lime Tomato Salad

Prep time: 10 minutes I **Cooking time:** 0 minutes I **Servings:** 4

Ingredients:
- 1 pound cherry tomatoes, halved
- 3 scallions, chopped
- 1 tablespoon olive oil
- A pinch of salt and black pepper
- 1 tablespoon lime juice
- ¼ cup parsley, chopped

Directions:
1. In a bowl, combine the tomatoes with the scallions and the other ingredients, toss and serve as a side salad.

Nutrition facts per serving: calories 180, fat 2, fiber 2, carbs 8, protein 6

Sage and Garlic Quinoa

Prep time: 10 minutes I **Cooking time:** 30 minutes I **Servings:** 4

Ingredients:
- 1 tablespoon olive oil
- 1 yellow onion, chopped
- 1 cup quinoa
- 2 cups chicken stock
- 1 tablespoon sage, chopped
- 2 garlic cloves, minced
- A pinch of salt and black pepper
- 1 tablespoon chives, chopped

Directions:
1. Heat up a pan with the oil over medium-high heat, add the onion and the garlic and sauté for 5 minutes.
2. Add the quinoa and the other ingredients, toss, cook over medium heat for 25 minutes more, divide between plates and serve.

Nutrition facts per serving: calories 182, fat 1, fiber 1, carbs 11, protein 8

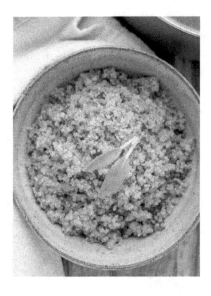

Chickpeas and Capers Salad

Prep time: 5 minutes I **Cooking time:** 0 minutes I **Servings:** 4

Ingredients:
- 2 cups chickpeas, cooked
- 1 tablespoon capers, chopped
- 2 tablespoons lime juice
- 2 tablespoons olive oil
- 4 spring onions, chopped
- 1 teaspoon chili powder
- 1 teaspoon cumin, ground
- 1 tablespoon parsley, chopped
- A pinch of salt and black pepper

Directions:
1. In a bowl, combine the chickpeas with the capers and the other ingredients, toss and serve as a side salad.

Nutrition facts per serving: calories 212, fat 4, fiber 4, carbs 12, protein 6

Quinoa and Green Beans

Prep time: 10 minutes I **Cooking time:** 30 minutes I **Servings:** 4

Ingredients:
- 1 tablespoon olive oil
- 1 yellow onion, chopped
- 1 cup quinoa
- ½ cup green beans, halved
- 2 cups chicken stock
- 2 garlic cloves, minced
- Salt and black pepper to the taste
- 1 tablespoon cilantro, chopped

Directions:
1. Heat up a pan with the olive oil over medium heat, add the onion and the garlic and sauté for 5 minutes.
2. Add the quinoa and the other ingredients, toss, bring to a simmer and cook over medium heat for 25 minutes.
3. Divide everything between plates and serve.

Nutrition facts per serving: calories 212, fat 1, fiber 2, carbs 2, protein 1

Cucumber Salad

Prep time: 5 minutes I **Cooking time:** 0 minutes I **Servings:** 4

Ingredients:
- 2 tablespoons olive oil
- 2 cucumbers, sliced
- 4 spring onions, chopped
- ½ cup cilantro, chopped
- ½ cup lemon juice
- Salt and black pepper to the taste

Directions:
1. In a salad bowl, combine the cucumbers with the spring onions and the other ingredients, toss and serve.

Nutrition facts per serving: calories 163, fat 1, fiber 2, carbs 7, protein 9

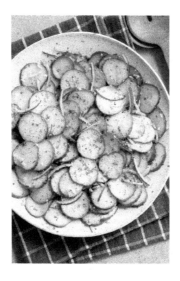

Balsamic Barley

Prep time: 5 minutes I **Cooking time:** 0 minutes I **Servings:** 4

Ingredients:
- 2 cups barley, cooked
- 1 cup baby kale
- 2 tablespoons almonds, chopped
- 2 tablespoons balsamic vinegar
- 1 tablespoon olive oil
- 1 tablespoon cilantro, chopped

Directions:
1. In a bowl, mix the barley with the kale, the almonds and the other ingredients, toss and serve as a side dish.

Nutrition facts per serving: calories 175, fat 3, fiber 3, carbs 5, protein 6

Mango and Spring Onions Mix

Prep time: 5 minutes I **Cooking time:** 0 minutes I **Servings:** 4

Ingredients:
- 2 mangos, peeled and chopped
- 2 spring onions, chopped
- 1 avocado, peeled, pitted and cubed
- 1 tablespoon olive oil
- 1 tablespoon chives, chopped
- 1 tablespoon oregano, chopped
- 1 tablespoon basil, chopped
- 2 tablespoons lemon juice
- Salt and black pepper to the taste

Directions:
1. In a salad bowl, mix the mangos with the spring onions, the avocado and the other ingredients, toss and serve as a side dish.

Nutrition facts per serving: calories 200, fat 5, fiber 7, carbs 12, protein 3

Cabbage and Dates Salad

Prep time: 10 minutes I **Cooking time:** 0 minutes I **Servings:** 4

Ingredients:
- 2 cups green cabbage, shredded
- 1 carrot, grated
- 4 dates, chopped
- 2 tablespoons walnuts, chopped
- 1 tablespoon lemon juice
- 2 garlic cloves, minced
- 1 tablespoon apple cider vinegar
- 3 tablespoons olive oil
- 1 tablespoon parsley, chopped
- A pinch of salt and black pepper

Directions:
1. In a bowl, combine the cabbage with the carrots, dates and the other ingredients, toss and serve as a side salad.

Nutrition facts per serving: calories 140, fat 3, fiber 4, carbs 5, protein 14

Orange Cucumber Salad

Prep time: 5 minutes I **Cooking time:** 0 minutes I **Servings:** 4

Ingredients:
- 2 cucumbers, sliced
- 1 green apple, cored and cubed
- 3 spring onions, chopped
- 3 tablespoons olive oil
- 4 teaspoons orange juice
- A pinch of salt and black pepper
- 1 tablespoon mint, chopped
- 1 tablespoon lemon juice

Directions:
1. In a bowl, mix the cucumbers with the apple, spring onions and the other ingredients, toss and serve as a side salad.

Nutrition facts per serving: calories 110, fat 0, fiber 3, carbs 6, protein 8

Lemon Avocado

Prep time: 5 minutes I **Cooking time:** 0 minutes I **Servings:** 4

Ingredients:
- 1 tablespoon olive oil
- 2 avocados, peeled, pitted and sliced
- 1 tablespoon parsley, chopped
- 1 tablespoon lemon juice
- 1 tablespoon lemon zest, grated
- A pinch of salt and black pepper

Directions:
1. In a bowl, combine the avocados with the oil, the parsley and the other ingredients, toss and serve as a side dish.

Nutrition facts per serving: calories 100, fat 0.5, fiber 1, carbs 5, protein 5

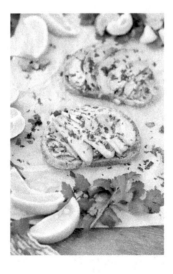

Almond Broccoli Mix

Prep time: 10 minutes I **Cooking time:** 20 minutes I **Servings:** 4

Ingredients:
- 2 endives, shredded
- 1 cup broccoli florets
- 2 tablespoons olive oil
- 1 tablespoon walnuts, chopped
- 1 tablespoon almonds, chopped
- 2 garlic cloves, minced
- 1 teaspoon rosemary, dried
- 1 teaspoon cumin, ground
- 1 teaspoon chili powder

Directions:
1. In a roasting pan, combine the endives with the broccoli and the other ingredients, toss and bake at 380 degrees F for 20 minutes.
2. Divide the mix between plates and serve.

Nutrition facts per serving: calories 139, fat 9.8, fiber 9.3, carbs 11.9, protein 4.9

Arugula and Tomato Salad

Prep time: 5 minutes I **Cooking time:** 0 minutes I **Servings:** 4

Ingredients:
- 2 cups baby arugula
- Juice of 1 lime
- ½ cup cherry tomatoes, halved
- 1 tablespoon olive oil
- 1 tablespoon balsamic vinegar
- A pinch of salt and black pepper
- 1 tablespoon chives, chopped

Directions:
1. In a salad bowl, mix the arugula with the lime juice, cherry tomatoes and the other ingredients, toss and serve.

Nutrition facts per serving: calories 190, fat 2, fiber 6, carbs 11, protein 7

Mint Tomatoes

Prep time: 10 minutes I **Cooking time:** 0 minutes I **Servings:** 4

Ingredients:
- 1 pound cherry tomatoes, halved
- 4 spring onions, chopped
- 2 tablespoons avocado oil
- 3 tablespoons mint, chopped
- A pinch of salt and black pepper
- 1 red chili pepper, chopped

Directions:
1. In a salad bowl, mix the tomatoes with the spring onions and the other ingredients, toss and serve as a side salad.

Nutrition facts per serving: calories 129, fat 3, fiber 2, carbs 8, protein 6

Radish and Spring Onions Salad

Prep time: 10 minutes I **Cooking time:** 0 minutes I **Servings:** 4

Ingredients:
- 2 cups radishes, sliced
- 2 spring onions, chopped
- A pinch of salt and black pepper
- 2 tablespoons balsamic vinegar
- 1 tablespoon chives, chopped
- 1 teaspoon rosemary, dried
- 2 tablespoons olive oil

Directions:
1. In a salad bowl, mix the radishes with the spring onions, salt, pepper and the other ingredients, toss and serve as a side salad.

Nutrition facts per serving: calories 110, fat 4, fiber 2, carbs 7, protein 7

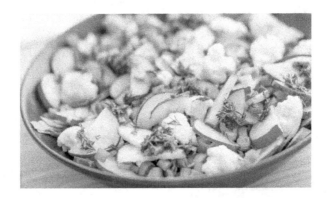

Garlic Green Beans and Okra

Prep time: 10 minutes I **Cooking time:** 30 minutes I **Servings:** 4

Ingredients:
1 cup okra, sliced
1 pound green beans, trimmed and halved
A pinch of salt and black pepper
3 scallions, chopped
2 garlic cloves, minced
3 tablespoons olive oil
1 tablespoon cilantro, chopped

Directions:
1. Spread the green beans and the okra on a baking sheet lined with parchment paper, add the rest of the ingredients, toss and bake at 360 degrees F for 30 minutes.
2. Divide the mix between plates and serve as a side dish.

Nutrition facts per serving: calories 120, fat 1, fiber 1, carbs 8, protein 7

Lemon and Chives Tomato Mix

Prep time: 10 minutes I **Cooking time:** 0 minutes I **Servings:** 4

Ingredients:
- 1 pound cherry tomatoes, halved
- 3 celery stalks, chopped
- 2 spring onions, chopped
- A pinch of sea salt and black pepper
- Juice of 1 lemon
- 1 tablespoon chives, chopped
- A pinch of cayenne pepper

Directions:
1. In a salad bowl, combine the cherry tomatoes with the celery and the other ingredients, toss and serve as a side dish.

Nutrition facts per serving: calories 80, fat 3, fiber 1, carbs 8, protein 5

Corn and Spinach Mix

Prep time: 10 minutes I **Cooking time:** 0 minutes I **Servings:** 4

Ingredients:
- 1 cup corn
- 1 avocado, peeled, pitted and cubed
- 1 tablespoon mint, chopped
- 1 cup baby spinach
- Juice of 1 lemon
- Zest of 1 lemon, grated
- 1 tablespoon avocado oil
- A pinch of sea salt and black pepper

Directions:
1. In a salad bowl, mix the corn with the avocado, the spinach and the other ingredients, toss and serve as a side dish.

Nutrition facts per serving: calories 90, fat 2, fiber 1, carbs 7, protein 5

Quinoa and Cucumber Mix

Prep time: 10 minutes I **Cooking time:** 0 minutes I **Servings:** 4

Ingredients:
- 1 cup quinoa, cooked
- 1 cup baby spinach
- A pinch of sea salt and black pepper
- 1 cucumber, chopped
- 1 teaspoon chili powder
- 2 tablespoons balsamic vinegar
- 2 tablespoons cilantro, chopped

Directions:
1. In a bowl, mix the quinoa with the spinach and the other ingredients, toss and serve as a side dish.

Nutrition facts per serving: calories 100, fat 0.5, fiber 2, carbs 6, protein 6

Mint and Lemon Asparagus

Prep time: 10 minutes I **Cooking time:** 10 minutes I **Servings:** 4

Ingredients:
- 1 pound asparagus, trimmed
- 2 tablespoons olive oil
- 3 garlic cloves, minced
- Salt and black pepper to the taste
- 1 teaspoon lemon zest, grated
- ¼ cup lemon juice
- ¼ cup mint leaves, chopped

Directions:
1. Heat up a pan with the oil over medium heat, add the garlic and sauté for 2 minutes.
2. Add the asparagus and the other ingredients, toss, cook for 8 minutes more, divide between plates and serve as a side dish.

Nutrition facts per serving: calories 100, fat 1, fiber 6, carbs 8, protein 6

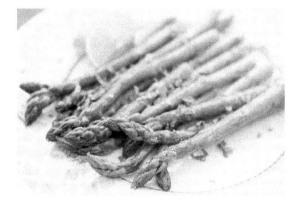

Chard and Spring Onions Mix

Prep time: 10 minutes I **Cooking time:** 15 minutes I **Servings:** 4

Ingredients:
- 2 spring onions, chopped
- 4 cups red chard, shredded
- 2 tablespoons olive oil
- 2 teaspoons ginger, grated
- ½ teaspoon red pepper flakes, crushed
- 2 tablespoons balsamic vinegar
- 1 tablespoon chives, chopped

Directions:
1. Heat up a pan with the oil over medium heat, add the spring onions and the ginger and sauté for 5 minutes.
2. Add the chard and the other ingredients, toss, cook for 10 minutes more, divide between plates and serve as a side dish.

Nutrition facts per serving: calories 160, fat 10, fiber 3, carbs 10, protein 5

Cabbage and Walnuts Mix

Prep time: 10 minutes I **Cooking time:** 0 minutes I **Servings:** 4

Ingredients:
- 1 cup green cabbage, shredded
- 1 cup tomatoes, cubed
- 2 tablespoons walnuts, chopped
- 1 bunch green onions, chopped
- ¼ cup balsamic vinegar
- 2 tablespoons olive oil
- 1 tablespoon chives, chopped
- A pinch of salt and black pepper

Directions:
1. In a salad bowl, mix the cabbage with the tomatoes, the walnuts and the other ingredients, toss and serve as a side dish.

Nutrition facts per serving: calories 140, fat 3, fiber 3, carbs 8, protein 6

Balsamic Carrots and Scallions Salad

Prep time: 10 minutes I **Cooking time:** 0 minutes I **Servings:** 4

Ingredients:
- 3 scallions, chopped
- 1 pound carrots, peeled and sliced
- ½ cup cilantro, chopped
- 3 tablespoons sesame seeds
- 2 tablespoons balsamic vinegar
- 2 tablespoons olive oil
- A pinch of salt and black pepper

Directions:
1. In a salad bowl, mix the carrots with the scallions and the other ingredients, toss well and serve as a side dish.

Nutrition facts per serving: calories 140, fat 4, fiber 3, carbs 5, protein 6

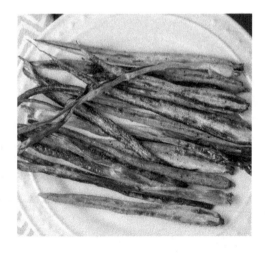

Sweet Potatoes and Walnuts Mix

Prep time: 10 minutes I **Cooking time:** 30 minutes I **Servings:** 4

Ingredients:
- 2 sweet potatoes, peeled and cut into wedges
- 2 tablespoons raisins
- 2 garlic cloves, minced
- 2 tablespoons walnuts, chopped
- Juice of ½ lemon
- 2 tablespoons olive oil
- A pinch of salt and black pepper

Directions:
1. In a roasting pan, combine the sweet potatoes with the raisins and the other ingredients, toss and bake at 370 degrees F for 30 minutes.
2. Divide everything between plates and serve.

Nutrition facts per serving: calories 120, fat 1, fiber 2, carbs 3, protein 5

Coconut Okra

Prep time: 10 minutes I **Cooking time:** 30 minutes I **Servings:** 4

Ingredients:
- 2 cups okra, sliced
- 1 teaspoon turmeric powder
- A pinch of salt and black pepper
- 1 teaspoon thyme, dried
- 2 tablespoons olive oil
- 1 tablespoon coconut aminos
- 1 tablespoon cilantro, chopped

Directions:
1. In a baking dish, combine the okra with the turmeric, salt, pepper and the other ingredients, toss and cook at 360 degrees F for 30 minutes.
2. Divide the mix between plates and serve as a side dish.

Nutrition facts per serving: calories 87, fat 7.2, fiber 1.8, carbs 5, protein 1

Coconut Green Beans

Prep time: 10 minutes I **Cooking time:** 30 minutes I **Servings:** 4

Ingredients:
- 1 pound green beans, trimmed and halved
- 2 tablespoons olive oil
- 2 garlic cloves, minced
- 1 yellow onion, chopped
- ½ cup coconut cream
- 1 teaspoon coriander, ground
- 1 teaspoon cumin, ground
- A pinch of red pepper flakes
- A pinch of salt and black pepper

Directions:
1. Heat up a pan with the oil over medium heat, add the onion and the garlic and sauté for 5 minutes.
2. Add the green beans and the other ingredients, toss, cook over medium heat for 25 minutes more, divide between plates and serve.

Nutrition facts per serving: calories 180, fat 14.5, fiber 5.2, carbs 13.1, protein 3.3

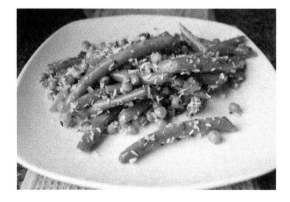

Radish Salad

Prep time: 10 minutes I **Cooking time:** 0 minutes I **Servings:** 4

Ingredients:
- 2 cups green cabbage, shredded
- ½ cup radishes, sliced
- 1 tablespoon olive oil
- 4 scallions, chopped
- A pinch of salt and black pepper
- 1 tablespoon chives, chopped
- 1 teaspoon sesame seeds

Directions:
1. In a bowl, combine the radishes with the cabbage and the other ingredients, toss and serve.

Nutrition facts per serving: calories 121, fat 3, fiber 4, carbs 8.30, protein 3

Paprika Beets and Chives

Prep time: 10 minutes I **Cooking time:** 40 minutes I **Servings:** 4

Ingredients:
- 1 pound red beets, peeled and roughly cubed
- 1 red onion, cut into wedges
- 1 tablespoon smoked paprika
- 1 teaspoon red pepper flakes, crushed
- 3 garlic cloves, minced
- A pinch of salt and black pepper
- 3 tablespoons olive oil
- 2 tablespoon chives, chopped

Directions:
1. In a baking dish, mix the beets with the onion, the paprika and the other ingredients, toss and bake at 380 degrees F for 40 minutes.
2. Divide everything between plates and serve as a side dish.

Nutrition facts per serving: calories 162, fat 4, fiber 7, carbs 11, protein 7

Roasted Rosemary Sprouts

Prep time: 5 minutes I **Cooking time:** 30 minutes I **Servings:** 4

Ingredients:
- 1 pound Brussels sprouts, trimmed and halved
- 2 carrots, grated
- 2 tablespoons avocado oil
- 1 tablespoon rosemary, chopped
- 2 tablespoons walnuts, chopped
- A pinch of salt and black pepper

Directions:
1. In a baking dish, mix the sprouts with the carrots, the oil and the other ingredients, toss and bake at 380 degrees F for 30 minutes.
2. Divide everything between plates and serve as a side dish.

Nutrition facts per serving: calories 191, fat 2, fiber 4, carbs 13, protein 7

Creamy Corn

Prep time: 10 minutes I **Cooking time:** 20 minutes I **Servings:** 4

Ingredients:
- 2 cups corn
- 2 cups cherry tomatoes, halved
- 1 cup coconut milk
- 1 tablespoon mint, chopped
- 1 teaspoon turmeric powder
- 1 teaspoon chili powder
- A pinch of salt and black pepper
- 2 tablespoons green onions, chopped

Directions:
1. In a pan, combine the corn with the cherry tomatoes, the milk and the other ingredients, toss, bring to a simmer and cook over medium heat for 20 minutes.
2. Divide the mix between plates and serve as a side dish.

Nutrition facts per serving: calories 199, fat 2, fiber 3, carbs 8, protein 6

Balsamic Squash Mix

Prep time: 10 minutes I **Cooking time:** 25 minutes I **Servings:** 4

Ingredients:
- 1 butternut squash, peeled and roughly cubed
- 2 spring onions, chopped
- 1 tablespoon avocado oil
- A pinch of salt and black pepper
- 1 tablespoon balsamic vinegar
- 1 tablespoon cilantro, chopped
- ½ cup pecans, toasted and chopped

Directions:
1. In a roasting pan, combine the squash with the spring onions and the other ingredients, toss and bake at 400 degrees F for 25 minutes.
2. Divide the mix between plates and serve.

Nutrition facts per serving: calories 211, fat 3, fiber 4, carbs 9, protein 6

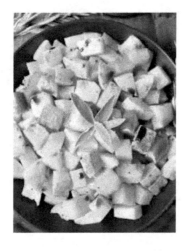

Cinnamon and Ginger Carrots Mix

Prep time: 10 minutes I **Cooking time:** 30 minutes I **Servings:** 4

Ingredients:
- 1 pound baby carrots, peeled
- 1 tablespoon ginger, grated
- 3 tablespoons cinnamon powder
- 1 tablespoon coconut oil, melted
- 1 tablespoon chives, chopped

Directions:
1. Spread the carrots on a baking sheet lined with parchment paper, add the ginger and the other ingredients, toss and bake at 380 degrees F for 30 minutes.
2. Divide everything between plates and serve.

Nutrition facts per serving: calories 198, fat 2, fiber 4, carbs 11, protein 6

Rice and Tomato Salad

Prep time: 10 minutes I **Cooking time:** 0 minutes I **Servings:** 4

Ingredients:
- 2 tablespoons olive oil
- 2 cups brown rice, cooked
- ½ cup cherry tomatoes, halved
- 2 teaspoons cumin, ground
- ¼ cup cilantro, chopped
- A pinch of salt and black pepper
- 2 tablespoons olive oil

Directions:
1. In a bowl, combine the rice with the oil and the other ingredients, toss and serve.

Nutrition facts per serving: calories 122, fat 4, fiber 3, carbs 8, protein 5

Curry and Lime Green Beans

Prep time: 10 minutes I **Cooking time:** 25 minutes I **Servings:** 4

Ingredients:
- 2 tablespoons olive oil
- 1 yellow onion, chopped
- 1 pound green beans, trimmed
- 2 teaspoons garlic, minced
- A pinch of salt and black pepper
- 2 teaspoons curry powder
- ½ cup vegetable stock
- ½ teaspoon brown mustard seeds
- 1 tablespoon lime juice

Directions:
1. Heat up a large pan with the oil over medium-high heat, add the onion and the garlic and sauté for 5 minutes.
2. Add the green beans and the other ingredients, toss, cook over medium heat for 20 minutes, divide between plates and serve.

Nutrition facts per serving: calories 181, fat 3, fiber 6, carbs 12, protein 6

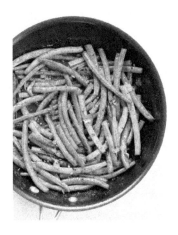

Chili Avocado and Onion Salad

Prep time: 10 minutes I **Cooking time:** 0 minutes I **Servings:** 4

Ingredients:
- 2 red onions, sliced
- 2 avocados, peeled, pitted and roughly sliced
- 1 tablespoon olive oil
- 1 tablespoon balsamic vinegar
- 1 tablespoon dill, chopped
- 1 teaspoon chili powder
- A pinch of salt and black pepper

Directions:
1. In a bowl, combine the avocado with the onions and the other ingredients, toss, and serve.

Nutrition facts per serving: calories 171, fat 2, fiber 7, carbs 13, protein 6

Hot Green Beans

Prep time: 10 minutes I **Cooking time:** 20 minutes I **Servings:** 4

Ingredients:
- 1 pound green beans, trimmed and halved
- 1 cup radishes, sliced
- 2 tablespoons olive oil
- 1 yellow onion, chopped
- A pinch of salt and black pepper
- 4 scallions, chopped
- 1 teaspoon chili flakes
- 1 tablespoon cilantro, chopped

Directions:
1. Heat up a pan with the oil over medium heat, add the onion and the scallions and sauté for 5 minutes.
2. Add the green beans and the other ingredients, toss, cook over medium heat for 15 minutes, divide between plates and serve.

Nutrition facts per serving: calories 60, fat 3, fiber 2, carbs 5, protein 1

Coriander Broccoli

Prep time: 10 minutes I **Cooking time:** 20 minutes I **Servings:** 4

Ingredients:
- 1 pound broccoli florets
- 1 cup green peas
- 1 teaspoon cumin, ground
- A pinch of salt and black pepper
- 1 tablespoon mint leaves, chopped
- 2 tablespoons olive oil
- 1 tablespoon coriander, chopped

Directions:
1. In a roasting pan, combine the broccoli with the peas, the mint and the other ingredients, toss and bake at 390 degrees F for 20 minutes.
2. Divide everything between plates and serve.

Nutrition facts per serving: calories 120, fat 6, fiber 1, carbs 5, protein 6

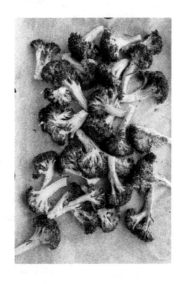

Garlic Bok Choy Mix

Prep time: 10 minutes I **Cooking time:** 20 minutes I **Servings:** 4

Ingredients:
- 1 pound bok choy, torn
- 1 yellow onion, chopped
- 1 tablespoon olive oil
- A pinch of salt and black pepper
- 1 tablespoon red pepper flakes, crushed
- 3 garlic cloves, minced
- ¼ cup cilantro, chopped

Directions:
1. Heat up a pan with the oil over medium heat, add the onion and the garlic and sauté for 5 minutes.
2. Add the bok choy and the other ingredients, toss, cook over medium heat for 15 minutes more, divide between plates and serve as a side dish.

Nutrition facts per serving: calories 143, fat 3, fiber 4, carbs 3, protein 6

Kale and Bok Choy Saute

Prep time: 5 minutes I **Cooking time:** 20 minutes I **Servings:** 4

Ingredients:
- 2 tablespoons olive oil
- 1 yellow onion, chopped
- 1 cup kale, torn
- 2 cups bok boy, torn
- 2 garlic cloves, minced
- 1 teaspoon turmeric powder
- 3 tablespoons lemon juice
- A pinch of salt and black pepper

Directions:
1. Heat up a pan with the oil over medium heat, add the onion and the garlic and sauté for 5 minutes.
2. Add the kale, bok choy and the other ingredients, toss, cook over medium heat for 15 minutes, divide between plates and serve.

Nutrition facts per serving: calories 180, fat 2, fiber 7, carbs 6, protein 8

Endives Salad

Prep time: 10 minutes I **Cooking time:** 0 minutes I **Servings:** 4

Ingredients:
- 2 endives, trimmed and thinly sliced
- 2 tablespoons olive oil
- 4 scallions, chopped
- 2 ounces watercress, chopped
- 1 tablespoon balsamic vinegar
- A pinch of salt and black pepper
- 1 tablespoon tarragon, chopped
- 1 tablespoon chives, chopped
- 1 tablespoon pine nuts, toasted
- 1 tablespoon walnuts, chopped

Directions:
1. In a bowl, mix the endives with the scallions, the watercress and the other ingredients, toss well and serve as a side salad.

Nutrition facts per serving: calories 140, fat 10.3, fiber 8.8, carbs 10.5, protein 4.8

Zucchini Saute

Prep time: 5 minutes I **Cooking time:** 20 minutes I **Servings:** 4

Ingredients:
- 1 cup kale, torn
- 2 zucchinis, sliced
- 1 yellow onion, chopped
- 2 tablespoons olive oil
- 1 teaspoon chili powder
- 1 teaspoon turmeric powder
- 1 tablespoon mint, chopped
- 1 tablespoon lemon juice
- A pinch of salt and black pepper

Directions:
1. Heat up a pan with the oil over medium heat, add the onion and sauté for 5 minutes.
2. Add the zucchinis, the kale and the other ingredients, toss, cook over medium heat for 15 minutes more, divide between plates and serve.

Nutrition facts per serving: calories 140, fat 1, fiber 2, carbs 11, protein 7

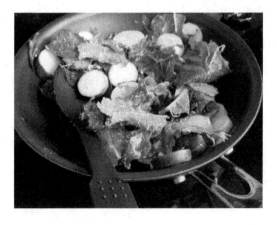

Cumin Corn Mix

Prep time: 10 minutes I **Cooking time:** 15 minutes I **Servings:** 4

Ingredients:
- 1 cup corn
- 2 zucchinis, roughly sliced
- 1 yellow onion, thinly sliced
- 2 tablespoon olive oil
- 2 teaspoons chili paste
- ¼ cup vegetable stock
- 1 tablespoon rosemary, chopped
- ½ teaspoon cumin, ground
- 4 green onions, chopped

Directions:
1. Heat up a pan with the oil over medium-high heat, add the onion and the chili paste, stir and sauté for 5 minutes
2. Add the corn, zucchinis and the other ingredients, toss well, cook over medium heat for 10 minutes more, divide between plates and serve as a side dish.

Nutrition facts per serving: calories 142, fat 7, fiber 4, carbs 5, protein 3

Spinach, Cucumber and Pine Nuts Salad

Prep time: 5 minutes I **Cooking time:** 0 minutes I **Servings:** 4

Ingredients:
- 1 pound baby spinach
- 1 cucumber, sliced
- 1 tomato, cubed
- 1 yellow onion, sliced
- 3 tablespoons olive oil
- ¼ cup pine nuts, toasted
- 2 tablespoons balsamic vinegar
- A pinch of salt and black pepper
- A pinch of red pepper, crushed

Directions:
1. In a bowl, combine the spinach with the cucumber, tomato and the other ingredients, toss and serve as a side salad.

Nutrition facts per serving: calories 120, fat 1, fiber 2, carbs 3, protein 6

Rosemary and Turmeric Endives

Prep time: 10 minutes I **Cooking time:** 20 minutes I **Servings:** 4

Ingredients:
- 2 endives, halved lengthwise
- 2 tablespoons olive oil
- 1 teaspoon rosemary, dried
- ½ teaspoon turmeric powder
- A pinch of black pepper

Directions:
1. In a baking pan, combine the endives with the oil and the other ingredients, toss gently, introduce in the oven and bake at 400 degrees F for 20 minutes.
2. Divide between plates and serve as a side dish.

Nutrition facts per serving: calories 66, fat 7.1, fiber 1, carbs 1.2, protein 0.3

Parmesan Endives

Prep time: 10 minutes I **Cooking time:** 20 minutes I **Servings:** 4

Ingredients:
- 4 endives, halved lengthwise
- 1 tablespoon lemon juice
- 1 tablespoon lemon zest, grated
- 2 tablespoons parmesan, grated
- 2 tablespoons olive oil
- A pinch of black pepper

Directions:
1. In a baking dish, combine the endives with the lemon juice and the other ingredients except the parmesan and toss.
2. Sprinkle the parmesan on top, bake the endives at 400 degrees F for 20 minutes, divide between plates and serve as a side dish.

Nutrition facts per serving: calories 71, fat 7.1, fiber 0.9, carbs 2.3, protein 0.9

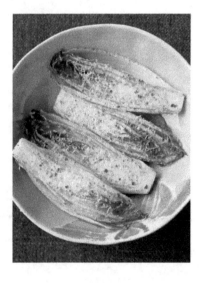

Pesto and Lemon Asparagus

Prep time: 10 minutes I **Cooking time:** 20 minutes I **Servings:** 4

Ingredients:
- 1 pound asparagus, trimmed
- 2 tablespoons basil pesto
- 1 tablespoon lemon juice
- A pinch of black pepper
- 3 tablespoons olive oil
- 2 tablespoons cilantro, chopped

Directions:
1. Arrange the asparagus n a lined baking sheet, add the pesto and the other ingredients, toss, introduce in the oven and cook at 400 degrees F for 20 minutes.
2. Divide between plates and serve as a side dish.

Nutrition facts per serving: calories 114, fat 10.7, fiber 2.4, carbs 4.6, protein 2.6

Paprika and Sesame Carrots

Prep time: 10 minutes I **Cooking time:** 30 minutes I **Servings:** 4

Ingredients:
- 1 pound baby carrots, trimmed
- 1 tablespoon sweet paprika
- 1 teaspoon lime juice
- 3 tablespoons olive oil
- A pinch of black pepper
- 1 teaspoon sesame seeds

Directions:
1. Arrange the carrots on a lined baking sheet, add the paprika and the other ingredients except the sesame seeds, toss, introduce in the oven and bake at 400 degrees F for 30 minutes.
2. Divide the carrots between plates, sprinkle sesame seeds on top and serve as a side dish.

Nutrition facts per serving: calories 142, fat 11.3, fiber 4.1, carbs 11.4, protein 1.2

Creamy Parmesan Potato

Prep time: 10 minutes I **Cooking time:** 1 hour I **Servings:** 8

Ingredients:
- 1 pound gold potatoes, peeled and cut into wedges
- 2 tablespoons olive oil
- 1 red onion, chopped
- 2 garlic cloves, minced
- 2 cups coconut cream
- 1 tablespoon thyme, chopped
- ¼ teaspoon nutmeg, ground
- ½ cup parmesan, grated

Directions:
1. Heat up a pan with the oil over medium heat, add the onion and the garlic and sauté for 5 minutes.
2. Add the potatoes and brown them for 5 minutes more.
3. Add the cream and the rest of the ingredients, toss gently, bring to a simmer and cook over medium heat for 40 minutes more.
4. Divide the mix between plates and serve as a side dish.

Nutrition facts per serving: calories 230, fat 19.1, fiber 3.3, carbs 14.3, protein 3.6

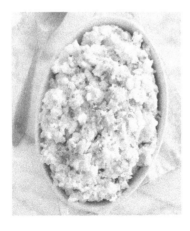

Cabbage Pan

Ingredients:
- 1 pound green cabbage, roughly shredded
- 2 tablespoons olive oil
- A pinch of black pepper
- 1 shallot, chopped
- 2 garlic cloves, minced
- 2 tablespoons balsamic vinegar
- 2 teaspoons hot paprika
- 1 teaspoon sesame seeds

Directions:
1. Heat up a pan with the oil over medium heat, add the shallot and the garlic and sauté for 5 minutes.
2. Add the cabbage and the other ingredients, toss, cook over medium heat for 15 minutes, divide between plates and serve.

Nutrition facts per serving: calories 101, fat 7.6, fiber 3.4, carbs 84, protein 1.9

Cilantro and Chili Broccoli

Prep time: 10 minutes I **Cooking time:** 30 minutes I **Servings:** 4

Ingredients:
- 2 tablespoons olive oil
- 1 pound broccoli florets
- 2 garlic cloves, minced
- 2 tablespoons chili sauce
- 1 tablespoon lemon juice
- A pinch of black pepper
- 2 tablespoons cilantro, chopped

Directions:
1. In a baking pan, combine the broccoli with the oil, garlic and the other ingredients, toss a bit, introduce in the oven and bake at 400 degrees F for 30 minutes.
2. Divide the mix between plates and serve as a side dish.

Nutrition facts per serving: calories 103, fat 7.4, fiber 3, carbs 8.3, protein 3.4

Mozzarella Brussels Sprouts

Prep time: 10 minutes I **Cooking time:** 25 minutes I **Servings:** 4

Ingredients:
- 1 tablespoon olive oil
- 1 pound Brussels sprouts, trimmed and halved
- 2 garlic cloves, minced
- ½ cup mozzarella, shredded
- A pinch of pepper flakes, crushed

Directions:
1. In a baking dish, combine the sprouts with the oil and the other ingredients except the cheese and toss.
2. Sprinkle the cheese on top, introduce in the oven and bake at 400 degrees F for 25 minutes.
3. Divide between plates and serve as a side dish.

Nutrition facts per serving: calories 91, fat 4.5, fiber 4.3, carbs 10.9, protein 5

Paprika Brussels Sprouts

Prep time: 10 minutes I **Cooking time:** 25 minutes I **Servings:** 4

Ingredients:
- 2 tablespoons olive oil
- 1 pound Brussels sprouts, trimmed and halved
- 3 green onions, chopped
- 2 garlic cloves, minced
- 1 tablespoon balsamic vinegar
- 1 tablespoon sweet paprika
- A pinch of black pepper

Directions:
1. In a baking pan, combine the Brussels sprouts with the oil and the other ingredients, toss and bake at 400 degrees F for 25 minutes.
2. Divide the mix between plates and serve.

Nutrition facts per serving: calories 121, fat 7.6, fiber 5.2, carbs 12.7, protein 4.4

Creamy Cauliflower Mash

Prep time: 10 minutes I **Cooking time:** 25 minutes I **Servings:** 4

Ingredients:
- 2 pounds cauliflower florets
- ½ cup coconut milk
- A pinch of black pepper
- ½ cup sour cream
- 1 tablespoon cilantro, chopped
- 1 tablespoon chives, chopped

Directions:
1. Put the cauliflower in a pot, add water to cover, bring to a boil over medium heat, cook for 25 minutes and drain.
2. Mash the cauliflower, add the milk, black pepper and the cream, whisk well, divide between plates, sprinkle the rest of the ingredients on top and serve.

Nutrition facts per serving: calories 188, fat 13.4, fiber 6.4, carbs 15, protein 6.1

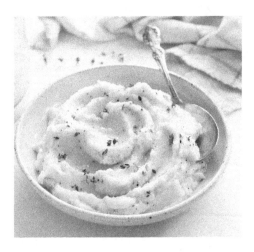

Avocado, Arugula and Olives Salad

Prep time: 5 minutes I **Cooking time:** 0 minutes I **Servings:** 4

Ingredients:
- 2 tablespoons olive oil
- 2 avocados, peeled, pitted and cut into wedges
- 1 cup kalamata olives, pitted and halved
- 1 cup tomatoes, cubed
- 1 tablespoon ginger, grated
- A pinch of black pepper
- 2 cups baby arugula
- 1 tablespoon balsamic vinegar

Directions:
1. In a bowl, combine the avocados with the kalamata and the other ingredients, toss and serve as a side dish.

Nutrition facts per serving: calories 320, fat 30.4, fiber 8.7, carbs 13.9, protein 3

Radish and Olives Salad

Prep time: 5 minutes I **Cooking time:** 0 minutes I **Servings:** 4

Ingredients:
- 2 green onions, sliced
- 1 pound radishes, cubed
- 2 tablespoons balsamic vinegar
- 2 tablespoon olive oil
- 1 teaspoon chili powder
- 1 cup black olives, pitted and halved
- A pinch of black pepper

Directions:
1. In a large salad bowl, combine radishes with the onions and the other ingredients, toss and serve as a side dish.

Nutrition facts per serving: calories 123, fat 10.8, fiber 3.3, carbs 7, protein 1.3

Lemony Endives and Cucumber Salad

Prep time: 5 minutes I **Cooking time:** 0 minutes I **Servings:** 4

Ingredients:
- 2 endives, roughly shredded
- 1 tablespoon dill, chopped
- ¼ cup lemon juice
- ¼ cup olive oil
- 2 cups baby spinach
- 2 tomatoes, cubed
- 1 cucumber, sliced
- ½ cups walnuts, chopped

Directions:
1. In a large bowl, combine the endives with the spinach and the other ingredients, toss and serve as a side dish.

Nutrition facts per serving: calories 238, fat 22.3, fiber 3.1, carbs 8.4, protein 5.7

Jalapeno Corn Mix

Prep time: 5 minutes I **Cooking time:** 0 minutes I **Servings:** 4

Ingredients:
- 2 tablespoons olive oil
- 1 tablespoon balsamic vinegar
- A pinch of black pepper
- 4 cups corn
- 2 cups black olives, pitted and halved
- 1 red onion, chopped
- ½ cup cherry tomatoes, halved
- 1 tablespoon basil, chopped
- 1 tablespoon jalapeno, chopped
- 2 cups romaine lettuce, shredded

Directions:
1. In a large bowl, combine the corn with the olives, lettuce and the other ingredients, toss well, divide between plates and serve as a side dish.

Nutrition facts per serving: calories 290, fat 16.1, fiber 7.4, carbs 37.6, protein 6.2

Arugula and Pomegranate Salad

Prep time: 5 minutes I **Cooking time:** 0 minutes I **Servings:** 4

Ingredients:
- ¼ cup pomegranate seeds
- 5 cups baby arugula
- 6 tablespoons green onions, chopped
- 1 tablespoon balsamic vinegar
- 2 tablespoons olive oil
- 3 tablespoons pine nuts
- ½ shallot, chopped

Directions:
1. In a salad bowl, combine the arugula with the pomegranate and the other ingredients, toss and serve.

Nutrition facts per serving: calories 120, fat 11.6, fiber 0.9, carbs 4.2, protein 1.8

Spinach Mix

Prep time: 10 minutes I **Cooking time:** 0 minutes I **Servings:** 4

Ingredients:
- 2 tablespoons olive oil
- 2 avocados, peeled, pitted and cut into wedges
- 3 cups baby spinach
- ¼ cup almonds, toasted and chopped
- 1 tablespoon lemon juice
- 1 tablespoon cilantro, chopped

Directions:
1. In a bowl, combine the avocados with the almonds, spinach and the other ingredients, toss and serve as a side dish.

Nutrition facts per serving: calories 181, fat 4, fiber 4.8, carbs 11.4, protein 6

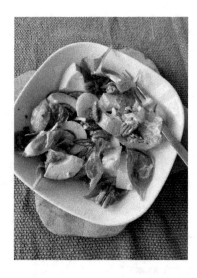

Green Beans and Lettuce Salad

Prep time: 4 minutes I **Cooking time:** 0 minutes I **Servings:** 4

Ingredients:
- Juice of 1 lime
- 2 cups romaine lettuce, shredded
- 1 cup corn
- ½ pound green beans, blanched and halved
- 1 cucumber, chopped
- 1/3 cup chives, chopped

Directions:
1. In a bowl, combine the green beans with the corn and the other ingredients, toss and serve.

Nutrition facts per serving: calories 225, fat 12, fiber 2.4, carbs 11.2, protein 3.5

Endives and Onion Salad

Prep time: 4 minutes I **Cooking time:** 0 minutes I **Servings:** 4

Ingredients:
- 3 tablespoons olive oil
- 2 endives, trimmed and shredded
- 2 tablespoons lime juice
- 1 tablespoon lime zest, grated
- 1 red onion, sliced
- 1 tablespoon balsamic vinegar
- 1 pound kale, torn
- A pinch of black pepper

Directions:
1. In a bowl, combine the endives with the kale and the other ingredients, toss well and serve cold as a side salad.

Nutrition facts per serving: calories 270, fat 11.4, fiber 5, carbs 14.3, protein 5.7

Garlic Edamame

Prep time: 5 minutes I **Cooking time:** 6 minutes I **Servings:** 4

Ingredients:
- 2 tablespoons olive oil
- 2 tablespoons balsamic vinegar
- 2 garlic cloves, minced
- 3 cups edamame, shelled
- 1 tablespoon chives, chopped
- 2 shallots, chopped

Directions:
1. Heat up a pan with the oil over medium heat, add the edamame, the garlic and the other ingredients, toss, cook for 6 minutes, divide between plates and serve.

Nutrition facts per serving: calories 270, fat 8.4, fiber 5.3, carbs 11.4, protein 6

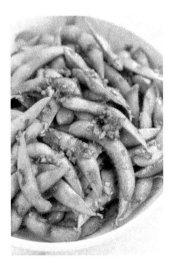

Grapes and Spinach Salad

Prep time: 5 minutes I **Cooking time:** 0 minutes I **Servings:** 4

Ingredients:
- 2 cups baby spinach
- 2 avocados, peeled, pitted and roughly cubed
- 1 cucumber, sliced
- 1 and ½ cups green grapes, halved
- 2 tablespoons avocado oil
- 1 tablespoon cider vinegar
- 2 tablespoons parsley, chopped
- A pinch of black pepper

Directions:
1. In a salad bowl, combine the baby spinach with the avocados and the other ingredients, toss and serve.

Nutrition facts per serving: calories 277, fat 11.4, fiber 5, carbs 14.6, protein 4

Parmesan Eggplant Mix

Prep time: 10 minutes I **Cooking time:** 20 minutes I **Servings:** 4

Ingredients:
- 2 big eggplants, roughly cubed
- 1 tablespoon oregano, chopped
- ½ cup parmesan, grated
- ¼ teaspoon garlic powder
- 2 tablespoons olive oil
- A pinch of black pepper

Directions:
1. In a baking pan combine the eggplants with the oregano and the other ingredients except the cheese and toss.
2. Sprinkle parmesan on top, introduce in the oven and bake at 370 degrees F for 20 minutes.
3. Divide between plates and serve as a side dish.

Nutrition facts per serving: calories 248, fat 8.4, fiber 4, carbs 14.3, protein 5.4

Parmesan Garlic Tomatoes Mix

Prep time: 10 minutes I **Cooking time:** 20 minutes I **Servings:** 4

Ingredients:
- 2 pounds tomatoes, halved
- 1 tablespoon basil, chopped
- 3 tablespoons olive oil
- Zest of 1 lemon, grated
- 3 garlic cloves, minced
- ¼ cup parmesan, grated
- A pinch of black pepper

Directions:
1. In a baking pan, combine the tomatoes with the basil and the other ingredients except the cheese and toss.
2. Sprinkle the parmesan on top, introduce in the oven at 375 degrees F for 20 minutes, divide between plates and serve as a side dish.

Nutrition facts per serving: calories 224, fat 12, fiber 4.3, carbs 10.8, protein 5.1

Parsley Mushrooms

Prep time: 10 minutes I **Cooking time:** 30 minutes I **Servings:** 4

Ingredients:
- 2 pounds white mushrooms, halved
- 4 garlic cloves, minced
- 2 tablespoons olive oil
- 1 tablespoon thyme, chopped
- 2 tablespoons parsley, chopped
- Black pepper to the taste

Directions:
1. In a baking pan, combine the mushrooms with the garlic and the other ingredients, toss, introduce in the oven and cook at 400 degrees F for 30 minutes.
2. Divide between plates and serve as a side dish.

Nutrition facts per serving: calories 251, fat 9.3, fiber 4, carbs 13.2, protein 6

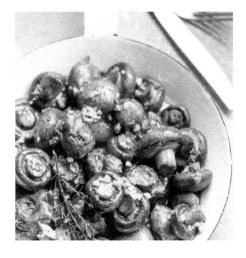

Spinach and Basil Sauté

Prep time: 10 minutes I **Cooking time:** 15 minutes I **Servings:** 4

Ingredients:
- 1 cup corn
- 1 pound spinach leaves
- 1 teaspoon sweet paprika
- 1 tablespoon olive oil
- 1 yellow onion, chopped
- ½ cup basil, torn
- A pinch of black pepper
- ½ teaspoon red pepper flakes

Directions:
1. Heat up a pan with the oil over medium-high heat, add the onion, stir and sauté for 5 minutes.
2. Add the corn, spinach and the other ingredients, toss, cook over medium heat for 10 minutes more, divide between plates and serve.

Nutrition facts per serving: calories 201, fat 13.1, fiber 2.5, carbs 14.4, protein 3.7

Corn and Shallots Mix

Prep time: 10 minutes I **Cooking time:** 15 minutes I **Servings:** 4

Ingredients:
- 4 cups corn
- 1 tablespoon avocado oil
- 2 shallots, chopped
- 1 teaspoon chili powder
- 2 tablespoons tomato pasta
- 3 scallions, chopped
- A pinch of black pepper

Directions:
1. Heat up a pan with the oil over medium-high heat, add the scallions and chili powder, stir and sauté for 5 minutes.
2. Add the corn and the other ingredients, toss, cook for 10 minutes more, divide between plates and serve as a side dish.

Nutrition facts per serving: calories 259, fat 11.1, fiber 2.6, carbs 13.2, protein 3.5

Spinach, Almonds and Capers Salad

Prep time: 10 minutes I **Cooking time:** 0 minutes I **Servings:** 4

Ingredients:
- 1 cup mango, peeled and cubed
- 4 cups baby spinach
- 1 tablespoon olive oil
- 2 spring onions, chopped
- 1 tablespoon lemon juice
- 1 tablespoon capers
- 1/3 cup almonds, chopped

Directions:
1. In a bowl, mix the spinach with the mango an d the other ingredients, toss and serve.

Nutrition facts per serving: calories 200, fat 7.4, fiber 3, carbs 4.7, protein 4.4

Mustard and Rosemary Potatoes

Prep time: 5 minutes I **Cooking time:** 1 hour I **Servings:** 4

Ingredients:
- 1 pound gold potatoes, peeled and cut into wedges
- 2 tablespoons olive oil
- A pinch of black pepper
- 2 tablespoons rosemary, chopped
- 1 tablespoon Dijon mustard
- 2 garlic cloves, minced

Directions:
1. In a baking pan, combine the potatoes with the oil and the other ingredients, toss, introduce in the oven at 400 degrees F and bake for about 1 hour.
2. Divide between plates and serve as a side dish right away.

Nutrition facts per serving: calories 237, fat 11.5, fiber 6.4, carbs 14.2, protein 9

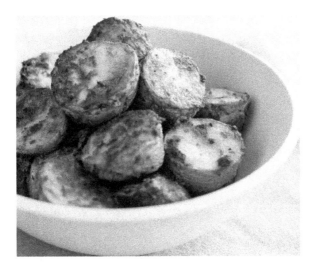

Cashew Brussels Sprouts

Prep time: 5 minutes I **Cooking time:** 30 minutes I **Servings:** 4

Ingredients:
- 1 pound Brussels sprouts, trimmed and halved
- 1 cup coconut cream
- 1 tablespoon olive oil
- 2 shallots, chopped
- A pinch of black pepper
- ½ cup cashews, chopped

Directions:
1. In a roasting pan, combine the sprouts with the cream and the rest of the ingredients, toss, and bake in the oven for 30 minutes at 350 degrees F.
2. Divide between plates and serve as a side dish.

Nutrition facts per serving: calories 270, fat 6.5, fiber 5.3, carbs 15.9, protein 3.4

Carrots and Onion Mix

Prep time: 10 minutes I **Cooking time:** 30 minutes I **Servings:** 4

Ingredients:
- 2 tablespoons olive oil
- 2 teaspoons sweet paprika
- 1 pound carrots, peeled and roughly cubed
- 1 red onion, chopped
- 1 tablespoon sage, chopped
- A pinch of black pepper

Directions:
1. In a baking pan, combine the carrots with the oil and the other ingredients, toss and bake at 380 degrees F for 30 minutes.
2. Divide between plates and serve.

Nutrition facts per serving: calories 200, fat 8.7, fiber 2.5, carbs 7.9, protein 4

Garlic Mushrooms

Prep time: 10 minutes I **Cooking time:** 20 minutes I **Servings:** 4

Ingredients:
- 1 pound white mushrooms, halved
- 2 cups corn
- 2 tablespoons olive oil
- 4 garlic cloves, minced
- 1 cup tomatoes, chopped
- A pinch of black pepper
- ½ teaspoon chili powder

Directions:
1. Heat up a pan with the oil over medium heat, add the mushrooms, garlic and the corn, stir and sauté for 10 minutes.
2. Add the rest of the ingredients, toss, cook over medium heat for 10 minutes more, divide between plates and serve.

Nutrition facts per serving: calories 285, fat 13, fiber 2.2, carbs 14.6, protein 6.7.

Pesto Green Beans

Prep time: 10 minutes I **Cooking time:** 15 minutes I **Servings:** 4

Ingredients:
- 2 tablespoons basil pesto
- 2 teaspoons sweet paprika
- 1 pound green beans, trimmed and halved
- Juice of 1 lemon
- 2 tablespoons olive oil
- 1 red onion, sliced
- A pinch of black pepper

Directions:
1. Heat up a pan with the oil over medium-high heat, add the onion, stir and sauté for 5 minutes.
2. Add the beans and the rest of the ingredients, toss, cook over medium heat for 10 minutes, divide between plates and serve.

Nutrition facts per serving: calories 280, fat 10, fiber 7.6, carbs 13.9, protein 4.7

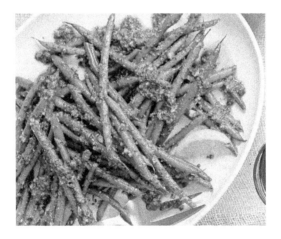

Tarragon and Lime Tomatoes

Prep time: 5 minutes I **Cooking time:** 0 minutes I **Servings:** 4

Ingredients:
- 1 and ½ tablespoon olive oil
- 1 pound tomatoes, cut into wedges
- 1 tablespoon lime juice
- 1 tablespoon lime zest, grated
- 2 tablespoons tarragon, chopped
- A pinch of black pepper

Directions:
1. In a bowl, combine the tomatoes with the other ingredients, toss and serve as a side salad.

Nutrition facts per serving: calories 170, fat 4, fiber 2.1, carbs 11.8, proteins 6

Parsley Beets

Prep time: 10 minutes I **Cooking time:** 30 minutes I **Servings:** 4

Ingredients:
- 4 beets, peeled and cut into wedges
- 3 tablespoons olive oil
- 2 tablespoons almonds, chopped
- 2 tablespoons balsamic vinegar
- A pinch of black pepper
- 2 tablespoons parsley, chopped

Directions:
1. In a baking pan, combine the beets with the oil and the other ingredients, toss, introduce in the oven and bake at 400 degrees F for 30 minutes.
2. Divide the mix between plates and serve.

Nutrition facts per serving: calories 230, fat 11, fiber 4.2, carbs 7.3, protein 3.6

Tomatoes and Vinegar Mix

Prep time: 5 minutes I **Cooking time:** 0 minutes I **Servings:** 4

Ingredients:
- 2 tablespoons mint, chopped
- 1 pound tomatoes, cut into wedges
- 2 cups corn
- 2 tablespoons olive oil
- 1 tablespoon rosemary vinegar
- A pinch of black pepper

Directions:
1. In a salad bowl, combine the tomatoes with the corn and the other ingredients, toss and serve.

Nutrition facts per serving: calories 230, fat 7.2, fiber 2, carbs 11.6, protein 4

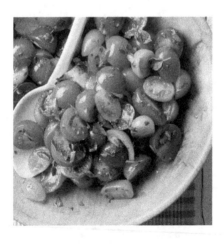

Zucchini Salsa

Prep time: 5 minutes I **Cooking time:** 10 minutes I **Servings:** 4

Ingredients:
- 2 tablespoons olive oil
- 2 zucchinis, cubed
- 1 avocado, peeled, pitted and cubed
- 2 tomatoes, cubed
- 1 cucumber, cubed
- 1 yellow onion, chopped
- 2 tablespoons fresh lime juice
- 2 tablespoons cilantro, chopped

Directions:
1. Heat up a pan with the oil over medium heat, add the onion and the zucchinis, toss and cook for 5 minutes.
2. Add the rest of the ingredients, toss, cook for 5 minutes more, divide between plates and serve.

Nutrition facts per serving: calories 290, fat 11.2, fiber 6.1, carbs 14.7, protein 5.6

Caraway Cabbage Mix

Prep time: 5 minutes I **Cooking time:** 0 minutes I **Servings:** 4

Ingredients:
- 2 green apples, cored and cubed
- 1 red cabbage head, shredded
- 2 tablespoons balsamic vinegar
- ½ teaspoon caraway seeds
- 2 tablespoons olive oil
- Black pepper to the taste

Directions:
1. In a bowl, combine the cabbage with the apples and the other ingredients, toss and serve as a side salad.

Nutrition facts per serving: calories 165, fat 7.4, fiber 7.3, carbs 26, protein 2.6

Baked Beets

Prep time: 10 minutes I **Cooking time:** 30 minutes I **Servings:** 4

Ingredients:
- 4 beets, peeled and cut into wedges
- 2 tablespoons olive oil
- 2 garlic cloves, minced
- A pinch of black pepper
- ¼ cup parsley, chopped
- ¼ cup walnuts, chopped

Directions:
1. In a baking dish, combine the beets with the oil and the other ingredients, toss to coat, introduce in the oven at 420 degrees F, bake for 30 minutes, divide between plates and serve as a side dish.

Nutrition facts per serving: calories 156, fat 11.8, fiber 2.7, carbs 11.5, protein 3.8

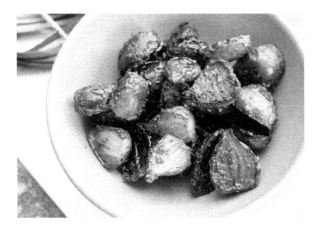

Dill Cabbage and Tomato

Prep time: 10 minutes I **Cooking time:** 15 minutes I **Servings:** 4

Ingredients:
- 1 pound green cabbage, shredded
- 1 yellow onion, chopped
- 1 tomato, cubed
- 1 tablespoon dill, chopped
- A pinch of black pepper
- 1 tablespoon olive oil

Directions:
1. Heat up a pan with the oil over medium heat, add the onion and sauté for 5 minutes.
2. Add the cabbage and the rest of the ingredients, toss, cook over medium heat for 10 minutes, divide between plates and serve.

Nutrition facts per serving: calories 74, fat 3.7, fiber 3.7, carbs 10.2, protein 2.1

Cabbage and Shallots Salad

Prep time: 5 minutes I **Cooking time:** 0 minutes I **Servings:** 4

Ingredients:
- 2 shallots, chopped
- 2 carrots, grated
- 1 big red cabbage head, shredded
- 1 tablespoon olive oil
- 1 tablespoon red vinegar
- A pinch of black pepper
- 1 tablespoon lime juice

Directions:
1. In a bowl, mix the cabbage with the shallots and the other ingredients, toss and serve as a side salad.

Nutrition facts per serving: calories 106, fat 3.8, fiber 6.5, carbs 18, protein 3.3

Tomato Salad

Prep time: 10 minutes I **Cooking time:** 0 minutes I **Servings:** 6

Ingredients:
- 1 pound cherry tomatoes, halved
- 2 tablespoons olive oil
- 1 cup kalamata olives, pitted and halved
- A pinch of black pepper
- 1 red onion, chopped
- 1 tablespoon balsamic vinegar
- ¼ cup cilantro, chopped

Directions:
1. In a bowl, mix the tomatoes with the olives and the other ingredients, toss and serve as a side salad.

Nutrition facts per serving: calories 131, fat 10.9, fiber 3.1, carbs 9.2, protein 1.6

Pesto Zucchini Salad

Prep time: 4 minutes I **Cooking time:** 0 minutes I **Servings:** 4

Ingredients:
- 2 zucchinis, cut with a spiralizer
- 1 red onion, sliced
- 1 tablespoon basil pesto
- 1 tablespoon lemon juice
- 1 tablespoon olive oil
- ½ cup cilantro, chopped
- Black pepper to the taste

Directions:
1. In a salad bowl, mix the zucchinis with the onion and the other ingredients, toss and serve.

Nutrition facts per serving: calories 58, fat 3.8, fiber 1.8, carbs 6, protein 1.6

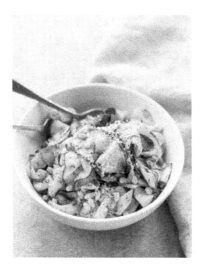

Carrots Slaw

Prep time: 4 minutes I **Cooking time:** 0 minutes I **Servings:** 4

Ingredients:
- 1 pound carrots, peeled and roughly grated
- 2 tablespoons avocado oil
- 2 tablespoons lemon juice
- 3 tablespoons sesame seeds
- ½ teaspoon curry powder
- 1 teaspoon rosemary, dried
- ½ teaspoon cumin, ground

Directions:
1. In a bowl, mix the carrots with the oil, lemon juice and the other ingredients, toss and serve cold as a side salad.

Nutrition facts per serving: calories 99, fat 4.4, fiber 4.2, carbs 13.7, protein 2.4

Lettuce Salad

Prep time: 5 minutes I **Cooking time:** 0 minutes I **Servings:** 4

Ingredients:
- 1 tablespoon ginger, grated
- 2 garlic cloves, minced
- 4 cups romaine lettuce, torn
- 1 beet, peeled and grated
- 2 green onions, chopped
- 1 tablespoon balsamic vinegar
- 1 tablespoon sesame seeds

Directions:
1. In a bowl, combine the lettuce with the ginger, garlic and the other ingredients, toss and serve as a side dish.

Nutrition facts per serving: calories 42, fat 1.4, fiber 1.5, carbs 6.7, protein 1.4

Chives Radishes

Prep time: 5 minutes I **Cooking time:** 0 minutes I **Servings:** 4

Ingredients:
- 1 pound red radishes, roughly cubed
- 1 tablespoon chives, chopped
- 1 tablespoon parsley, chopped
- 1 tablespoon oregano, chopped
- 2 tablespoons olive oil
- 1 tablespoon lime juice
- Black pepper to the taste

Directions:
1. In a salad bowl, mix the radishes with the chives and the other ingredients, toss and serve.

Nutrition facts per serving: calories 85, fat 7.3, fiber 2.4, carbs 5.6, protein 1

Lime Fennel Mix

Prep time: 5 minutes I **Cooking time:** 20 minutes I **Servings:** 4

Ingredients:
- 2 fennel bulbs, sliced
- 1 teaspoon sweet paprika
- 1 small red onion, sliced
- 2 tablespoons olive oil
- 2 tablespoons lime juice
- 2 tablespoons dill, chopped
- Black pepper to the taste

Directions:
1. In a roasting pan, combine the fennel with the paprika and the other ingredients, toss, and bake at 380 degrees F for 20 minutes.
2. Divide the mix between plates and serve.

Nutrition facts per serving: calories 114, fat 7.4, fiber 4.5, carbs 13.2, protein 2.1

Oregano Peppers

Prep time: 10 minutes I **Cooking time:** 30 minutes I **Servings:** 4

Ingredients:
- 1 pound mixed bell peppers, cut into wedges
- 1 red onion, thinly sliced
- 2 tablespoons olive oil
- Black pepper to the taste
- 1 tablespoon oregano, chopped
- 2 tablespoons mint leaves, chopped

Directions:
1. In a roasting pan, combine the bell peppers with the onion and the other ingredients, toss and bake at 380 degrees F for 30 minutes.
2. Divide the mix between plates and serve.

Nutrition facts per serving: calories 240, fat 8.2, fiber 4.2, carbs 11.3, protein 5.6

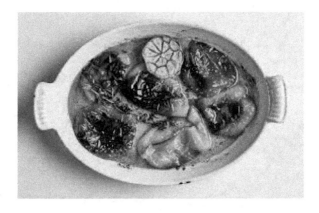

Red Cabbage Sauté

Prep time: 5 minutes I **Cooking time:** 15 minutes I **Servings:** 4

Ingredients:
- 1 pound red cabbage, shredded
- 8 dates, pitted and sliced
- 2 tablespoons olive oil
- ¼ cup veggie stock
- 2 tablespoons chives, chopped
- 2 tablespoons lemon juice
- Black pepper to the taste

Directions:
1. Heat up a pan with the oil over medium heat, add the cabbage and the dates, toss and cook for 4 minutes.
2. Add the stock and the other ingredients, toss, cook over medium heat for 11 minutes more, divide between plates and serve.

Nutrition facts per serving: calories 280, fat 8.1, fiber 4.1, carbs 8.7, protein 6.3

Black Beans and Shallots Mix

Prep time: 4 minutes I **Cooking time:** 0 minutes I **Servings:** 4

Ingredients:
- 3 cups black beans, cooked
- 1 cup cherry tomatoes, halved
- 2 shallots, chopped
- 3 tablespoons olive oil
- 1 tablespoon balsamic vinegar
- Black pepper to the taste
- 1 tablespoon chives, chopped

Directions:
1. In a bowl, combine the beans with the tomatoes and the other ingredients, toss and serve cold as a side dish.

Nutrition facts per serving: calories 310, fat 11.0, fiber 5.3, carbs 19.6, protein 6.8

Cilantro Olives Mix

Prep time: 4 minutes I **Cooking time:** 0 minutes I **Servings:** 4

Ingredients:
- 2 spring onions, chopped
- 2 endives, shredded
- 1 cup black olives, pitted and sliced
- ½ cup kalamata olives, pitted and sliced
- ¼ cup apple cider vinegar
- 2 tablespoons olive oil
- 1 tablespoons cilantro, chopped

Directions:
1. In a bowl, mix the endives with the olives and the other ingredients, toss and serve.

Nutrition facts per serving: calories 230, fat 9.1, fiber 6.3, carbs 14.6, protein 7.2

Basil Tomatoes and Cucumber Mix

Prep time: 5 minutes I **Cooking time:** 0 minutes I **Servings:** 4

Ingredients:
- ½ pound tomatoes, cubed
- 2 cucumber, sliced
- 1 tablespoon olive oil
- 2 spring onions, chopped
- Black pepper to the taste
- Juice of 1 lime
- ½ cup basil, chopped

Directions:
1. In a salad bowl, combine the tomatoes with the cucumber and the other ingredients, toss and serve cold.

Nutrition facts per serving: calories 224, fat 11.2, fiber 5.1, carbs 8.9, protein 6.2

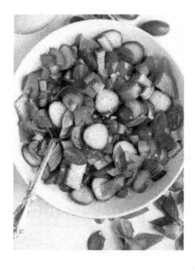

Peppers Salad

Prep time: 5 minutes I **Cooking time:** 0 minutes I **Servings:** 4

Ingredients:
- 1 cup cherry tomatoes, halved
- 1 yellow bell pepper, chopped
- 1 red bell pepper, chopped
- 1 green bell pepper, chopped
- ½ pound carrots, shredded
- 3 tablespoons red wine vinegar
- 2 tablespoons olive oil
- 1 tablespoon cilantro, chopped
- Black pepper to the taste

Directions:
1. In a salad bowl, mix the tomatoes with the peppers, carrots and the other ingredients, toss and serve as a side salad.

Nutrition facts per serving: calories 123, fat 4, fiber 8.4, carbs 14.4, protein 1.1

Thyme Rice Mix

Prep time: 10 minutes I **Cooking time:** 30 minutes I **Servings:** 4

Ingredients:
- 2 tablespoons olive oil
- 1 yellow onion, chopped
- 1 cup black beans, cooked
- 2 cup black rice
- 4 cups chicken stock
- 2 tablespoons thyme, chopped
- Zest of ½ lemon, grated
- A pinch of black pepper

Directions:
1. Heat up a pan with the oil over medium-high heat, add the onion, stir and sauté for 4 minutes.
2. Add the beans, rice and the other ingredients, toss, bring to a boil and cook over medium heat for 25 minutes.
3. Stir the mix, divide between plates and serve.

Nutrition facts per serving: calories 290, fat 15.3, fiber 6.2, carbs 14.6, protein 8

Rice and Cranberries Mix

Prep time: 10 minutes I **Cooking time:** 25 minutes I **Servings:** 4

Ingredients:
- 1 cup cauliflower florets
- 1 cup brown rice
- 2 cups chicken stock
- 1 tablespoon avocado oil
- 2 shallots, chopped
- ¼ cup cranberries
- ½ cup almonds, sliced

Directions:
1. Heat up a pan with the oil over medium heat, add the shallots, stir and sauté for 5 minutes.
2. Add the cauliflower, the rice and the other ingredients, toss, bring to a simmer and cook over medium heat for 20 minutes.
3. Divide the mix between plates and serve.

Nutrition facts per serving: calories 290, fat 15.1, fiber 5.6, carbs 7, protein 4.5

Oregano Beans Salad

Prep time: 10 minutes I **Cooking time:** 0 minutes I **Servings:** 4

Ingredients:
- 2 cups black beans, cooked
- 2 cups white beans, cooked
- 2 tablespoons balsamic vinegar
- 2 tablespoons olive oil
- 1 teaspoon oregano, dried
- 1 teaspoon basil, dried
- 1 tablespoon chives, chopped

Directions:
1. In a salad bowl, combine the beans with the vinegar and the other ingredients, toss and serve as a side salad.

Nutrition facts per serving: calories 322, fat 15.1, fiber 10, carbs 22.0, protein 7

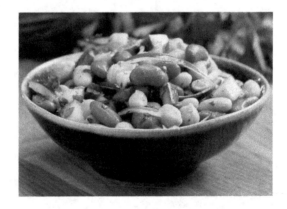

Coconut Beets

Prep time: 5 minutes I **Cooking time:** 20 minutes I **Servings:** 4

Ingredients:
- 1 pound beets, peeled and cubed
- 1 red onion, chopped
- 1 tablespoon olive oil
- ½ cup coconut cream
- 4 tablespoons non-fat yogurt
- 1 tablespoon chives, chopped

Directions:
1. Heat up a pan with the oil over medium heat, add the onion, stir and sauté for 4 minutes.
2. Add the beets, cream and the other ingredients, toss, cook over medium heat for 15 minutes more, divide between plates and serve.

Nutrition facts per serving: calories 250, fat 13.4, fiber 3, carbs 13.3, protein 6.4

Avocado Mix

Prep time: 10 minutes I **Cooking time:** 14 minutes I **Servings:** 4

Ingredients:
- 1 tablespoon avocado oil
- 1 teaspoon sweet paprika
- 1 pound mixed bell peppers, cut into strips
- 1 avocado, peeled, pitted and halved
- 1 teaspoon garlic powder
- 1 teaspoon rosemary, dried
- ½ cup veggie stock
- Black pepper to the taste

Directions:
1. Heat up a pan with the oil over medium-high heat, add all the bell peppers, stir and sauté for 5 minutes.
2. Add the rest of the ingredients, toss, cook for 9 minutes more over medium heat, divide between plates and serve.

Nutrition facts per serving: calories 245, fat 13.8, fiber 5, carbs 22.5, protein 5.4

Roasted Sweet Potato

Prep time: 10 minutes I **Cooking time:** 1 hour I **Servings:** 4

Ingredients:
- 3 tablespoons olive oil
- 2 sweet potatoes, peeled and cut into wedges
- 2 beets, peeled, and cut into wedges
- 1 tablespoon oregano, chopped
- 1 tablespoon lime juice
- Black pepper to the taste

Directions:
1. Arrange the sweet potatoes and the beets on a lined baking sheet, add the rest of the ingredients, toss, introduce in the oven and bake at 375 degrees F for 1 hour/
2. Divide between plates and serve as a side dish.

Nutrition facts per serving: calories 240, fat 11.2, fiber 4, carbs 8.6, protein 12.1

Coconut Kale Sauté

Prep time: 10 minutes I **Cooking time:** 15 minutes I **Servings:** 4

Ingredients:
- 2 tablespoons olive oil
- 3 tablespoons coconut aminos
- 1 pound kale, torn
- 1 red onion, chopped
- 2 garlic cloves, minced
- 1 tablespoon lime juice
- 1 tablespoon cilantro, chopped

Directions:
1. Heat up a pan with the olive oil over medium heat, add the onion and the garlic and sauté for 5 minutes.
2. Add the kale and the other ingredients, toss, cook over medium heat for 10 minutes, divide between plates and serve.

Nutrition facts per serving: calories 200, fat 7.1, fiber 2, carbs 6.4, protein 6

Allspice Carrots

Prep time: 10 minutes I **Cooking time:** 20 minutes I **Servings:** 4

Ingredients:
- 1 tablespoon lemon juice
- 1 tablespoon olive oil
- ½ teaspoon allspice, ground
- ½ teaspoon cumin, ground
- ½ teaspoon nutmeg, ground
- 1 pound baby carrots, trimmed
- 1 tablespoon rosemary, chopped
- Black pepper to the taste

Directions:
1. In a roasting pan, combine the carrots with the lemon juice, oil and the other ingredients, toss, introduce in the oven and bake at 400 degrees F for 20 minutes.
2. Divide between plates and serve.

Nutrition facts per serving: calories 260, fat 11.2, fiber 4.5, carbs 8.3, protein 4.3

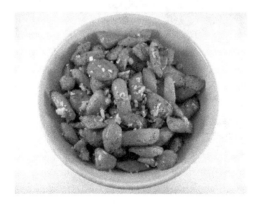

Lemony Dill Artichokes

Prep time: 10 minutes I **Cooking time:** 20 minutes I **Servings:** 4

Ingredients:
- 2 tablespoons lemon juice
- 4 artichokes, trimmed and halved
- 1 tablespoon dill, chopped
- 2 tablespoons olive oil
- A pinch of black pepper

Directions:
1. In a roasting pan, combine the artichokes with the lemon juice and the other ingredients, toss gently and bake at 400 degrees F for 20 minutes. Divide between plates and serve.

Nutrition facts per serving: calories 140, fat 7.3, fiber 8.9, carbs 17.7, protein 5.5

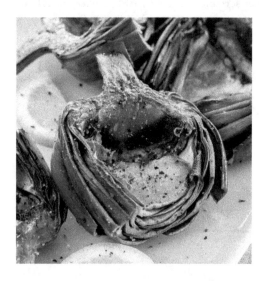

CPSIA information can be obtained
at www.ICGtesting.com
Printed in the USA
LVHW020103040121
675552LV00011B/460

9 781801 479707